Fifteen Minutes
with You

Fifteen Minutes with You

with You

Making the most of 'The Consultation'

Dr Andy Hershon

Introduction

So where on earth do I start? I'm a 55-year-old GP sitting in front of my slightly unreliable laptop with the vague thought of writing a book. I've dangled a few words out on to Twitter, and a fair few suggested I give it a go. I really hope they were serious and not just being 'nice'...

My plan is to enthuse you with my long-term passion for primary care, and more specifically to give you my personal insights into what I believe to be the very essence of general practice, 'The Consultation'. When Morrissey back in 1984 (sadly my era) waxed lyrical in the song 'Reel around the Fountain' about 'Fifteen Minutes with You' I doubt he had any thoughts that down the line a middle-aged bloke would use his words as inspiration for a book vaguely about medicine.

The fifteen minutes I shall be discussing are incredibly important and potentially life-changing to every patient that comes our way as clinicians. What an honour and a privilege it is to be given the chance to change such lives on a day-to-day basis. Surely no job could be as fulfilling; I have been in general practice for thirty years, and I've never for one minute been bored. For our part, I think we ought to be doing our utmost to perform our best in every single consultation, such is the trust put in us.

So who am I to tell you what you should be doing? Well, I'm no one, really. I've no doctorate in 'The Consultation', but I've been doing it a fair while and I have got a good deal of experience in what works. No way am I telling you what to do, anyway; I'm simply sharing my outlook and ways of doing things with you to reflect on. As I have told numerous students over the years, feel free to take what you want from the way I consult, but also feel free to reject parts you feel you might already do better. You'll have no doubt already read or learnt about 'The Consultation', and may suggest that what I'm writing is similar to all the others (Neighbour, Pendleton et al), and you'd probably be right. After all, each of us probably welcomes the patient in our own way, gets stuck into the nitty-gritty of the consultation, and then sums up. What I hope to do, as well as entertain you, is look at how I feel the potential of the fifteen minutes can be maximised, and how external factors may be involved and used to make the said consultation more effective.

My suggestions are not solely for GPs, although that is obviously the area in which I have gained my expertise. Thirty years ago when I started in Practice, we were the only ones carrying out consultations. Now, however, the landscape has changed completely. So many healthcare professionals are now carrying out consultations; in our surgery we have practice nurses who are the mainstay of chronic disease management, and advanced practitioners who are addressing acute care and doing most of our visits. We have pharmacists attached to our surgeries doing medication reviews, and also getting involved in long-term care. I would like to think that all those whose job it is to draw out health information and act on it might benefit from looking at some of the ideas I will be offering in the forthcoming pages.

So who am I?

I'm a little wary at the moment. I've read dozens of autobiographies where the famous footballer or actor tells me at length about sitting in their grandparents' house with their brothers and sisters, which school they went to and even what their mother gave them for tea on Sundays. I'm seriously not interested; I want to know about the big games, the other movie stars and hear the witty anecdotes – the reasons why I actually bought the book. I'll give you a brief insight into how I ended up here, but feel free to move forward in the book. I won't hold it against you...much.

Believe it or not, I was a linguist at school, particularly enjoying French, Latin and German. I actually think having a broad skill mix including, dare I say, a background in the 'Arts' is a strength rather than a weakness. My feelings have always been that to be a good GP you need sound scientific knowledge which should be applied with the communicative brush of an artist. I always fancied being a doctor (once I realised I wasn't good enough to play for Liverpool...), and from the age of twelve I was driven. It sounded so exciting: using your magical knowledge to help people every day and all that. I was right, and have never regretted that decision for a single moment.

I left my home town of Liverpool aged seventeen to start my medical course at Manchester University. How young lives are planned. The thought of leaving my family home, but being close enough to get back for my beloved Liverpool Football Club games, really appealed. I still think it was a top decision, although how I reached it was more than a little circumspect!

I loved medical school, and always thought that my future lay in general practice. I think my rationale was around being the best option to help most folk in the time available. It rankled with me then, and still does now, when people think of general practice as being a choice made only when options of being a consultant aren't available. I *am* a consultant, a consultant in primary care, thank you very much!

Before 'settling down' into any long-term job, I travelled a little (Jersey and Australia), and spent a few years in the field of psychiatry; being psychiatric registrar in Jersey was a nice little number. Mental health has always been a love of mine, and a primary care setting seemed the ideal opportunity to improve the mental wellbeing of those in the community. Many GPs are nervous around treating mental illness. Poor hospital-based undergraduate training and lack of time is a real issue. I think we can however make a good fist of it, and later in the book I'll give you my thoughts on how I think this can be done.

Eventually I did my GP training, and chanced upon a job straight after the end of my training year in Hattersley, a deprived overflow estate on the east side of Manchester. My trainer's wife worked in Hattersley, and I initially worked as a locum there. Sadly, she passed away, and as I seemed to fit in pretty well, I was offered the chance to join the partnership.

I felt at home immediately. They were, and continue to be, the sort of down-to-earth people I love to deal with. That was in 1991, and I am still enjoying life on 'The Estate' twenty-nine years later. I have always felt welcome, and have joined so many patient groups over the years. I've sat on the local housing committee as a guest, joined support meetings, gone on patient group walks. Keeping an eye on local resources in our community and being a part of these resources has been fulfilling, but also useful for my patients. I've always seen my role as a GP as a holistic one. If ten minutes of my time can make a difference to a patient, it's worth doing; whether that involves making elderly patients sandwiches, or even taking their dogs for a walk, I've been up for it over the years.

In days gone by I even chatted to my patients in the local bookmakers! You may well ask what a supposed upstanding pillar of society is doing standing against a pillar at the bookies, but no one seemed to mind. In fact it seemed to work the other way, being perceived as 'one of them'. A good few times they overestimated my powers. "Who's going to win, doc?" I was asked. "Ladbrokes," I generally replied...

I remember fondly organising football matches on the local pitch near my surgery. I took my children to play, and before I knew it, groups of young footballers appeared expecting me to organise a match, and obviously I couldn't let them down! This went on for several years. Sadly, when they grew up my lads started organising their own games and old Dad was left stranded! Some of these youngsters still come to see me, and fondly reminisce about these games. They have now grown up, many with their own children. Knowing so much about the 'goings on' on the estate, as well as a deep knowledge of the families thereon is rewarding, and an incredibly useful background to many consultations. It gives me, in a way, a head start in many consultations, something I believe to be so important in fulfilling a consultation's potential.

'Getting a head start'

The time we have with each patient is limited; otherwise we wouldn't be able to serve the large numbers that we do. While fifteen minutes is so much better than the five-minute consultations we had when I first started, it is still somewhat challenging. We have so much to do. We might be expected to treat the 'presenting problem', or even problems. There may be QOF alerts ('Quality Outcomes Framework' is a way in which we reach certain quality targets, and get part of our income as a consequence). They might need a medication review (NOT a box ticking exercise! – a hobby horse I'll come back to at some stage!). I might need to look at their underlying chronic diseases. I may even find an unannounced depressive disorder I'd be keen not to miss.

I've already got some sort of head start as I mentioned in the introduction. So many adults come in on whom I did six-week baby checks so many years ago. They may also remember me treating their ear infections when they were young. I probably know their parents, and they may remember that I was at the house daily when their grandmother breathed her last, hopefully without pain or anxiety. Not only do I know many members of the family, but often I'm also aware of family dynamics. All this hopefully builds trust in the upcoming consultation. It's certainly not a prerequisite – how can it be? Happily not all GPs are aged fifty-five with thirty years' experience, but it certainly helps.

There are other ways to get some sort of head start. If possible, having some idea of the issues which might be raised can be very useful. There may be something written in the appointment slot by whoever booked the appointment. It's worth taking a look, without being too led by what's been entered.

I often steal a couple of my fifteen minutes to look into the recent and past record. Patients tend to think you automatically know what's in their past histories, that you have intimate knowledge of every letter that refers to them. Sadly I can't offer that, but having a solid idea of what they've been through reaps rewards early in the consultation. Alternatively, having no clue can leave you as the GP in a difficult situation, with the patient feeling slightly wary that they're speaking to a total stranger. We all love 'continuity of care'; as GPs we tend to know instinctively what we were thinking 'last time,' so can move forward more successfully. For the patient this continuity gives reassurance that they are speaking to someone previously involved with their case, knowing the intricacies therein. We know that this isn't always possible, and often reassure that 'it's all in the records so Dr X (the doctor seeing the patient next) will know'. I think we owe it to the patient to make sure that to some extent this is true, and that if we have thoughts or plans we should adequately document them.

A little tip: if you are going to spend time going back through the records to clarify various details, it's probably a good idea to put what you have found at the top of the record where it is easily visible and accessible. Your hard work this time won't be duplicated next time the patient comes in, and if it's not yourself seeing them again, your colleague will be pretty thankful to you for helping them gain further knowledge about the patient easily. If you're feeling particularly keen, why not take the opportunity to clean up the summary a little? I spent some time in the past as CCG IT lead looking at 'active problem' lists and summaries. Most summaries weren't too bad, although there were plenty of 'had a chat' as active issues; some, however, were pretty poor! My ideal 'problem' summary is one which gives you the main issues in current and past history in a fairly quick glimpse: something you wouldn't be embarrassed about if it were seen by a secondary care colleague who had never seen the patient. I've seen times when there was so much trivia on the massive problem list that 'seeing the wood for the trees' had become a serious issue. I like a good tidy-up (not at home, I hear my wife saying in the background – and she's right!).

One area where I'd suggest the 'head start' is essential is prior to visiting patients in the community. They are often the most ill with multiple comorbidities. Most of us go out with a printed brief summary rather than having the full records to hand. It's so important to have a good peruse of the records before leaving the practice, and hopefully a decent quality summary to take out with you. Without this prior knowledge you will be entering that particular consultation at a disadvantage, and generally might not do the patient justice.

I sometimes prepare for the next consultation's 'head start' by putting the odd line in the record. Just little things to show you know about them, and that you care. If they're going abroad, I tend to note where to. I like to know how their work's going and the names and ages of their children, even. The one thing I don't need to note is their football allegiances! My Liverpool poster is generally a talking point (especially as I work in Manchester!) and I seem to have a special part of my brain given to football banter. I've occasionally wished their team, and my team's rival, well in the next game – they know I don't mean it.

Joking aside... it helps, I think, to know some small things about the patient. Many a consultation has started with: "How was Wales?", "Is Jack doing okay in school?", or even "Your team did well on Saturday". It seems to put folk at ease before allowing me to hear about their deepest fears.

At this point I'm going to mention the presence of the Computer, our trusty saver of our data.

Computers in General Practice

I came from an era when there were no computers. No keyboards, no QOF alerts. Let's be honest, though; they are a force for good. I have no time for nostalgia, for 'the good old days'. Those days often meant illegible record keeping, five-minute appointments, missed follow-up of long-term conditions and poor medicines management. I occasionally look back at written records, and I'm actually shocked by how awful they were. When I was a 'trainee', as it was called then in 1990, computers were just starting to become the 'norm'. One member of the practice refused point blank to have a computer. There was almost a pride in his refusal – "I'm a good GP without it, why should I start now?". I think to be honest, he was a little scared of feeling helpless. I had just bought a computer at home. It was a far cry from today's offerings; my computer had a fraction of the power of my current mobile phone. Talking of mobile phones, I didn't see one of them until 1989 when my group of psychiatry juniors in Jersey hired one, and very large it was, so we could do our 'on-call' from the beach, or occasionally the local pub or night club! I vividly remember doing a GP locum in the early nineties for a local colleague. Being computer literate, as I liked to think I was, I asked the staff to turn on his system. Neither the GP staff nor the GP hiring me had any idea how to actually switch the thing on. I presume it must have been a freebee from the FHSA (Family Health Service Authority) as it was then. They certainly weren't the absolute necessity that they are now. Most of us in the very early days kept two sets of notes. We wrote on screen, but we also wrote in the Lloyd George files we now see locked away in cupboards. I think it was just in case the computer blew up and all the data would be lost. Ironically, it was far more frequent for the written notes to be lost completely; a bit like what happens sometimes in hospitals to this day: "I saw this patient in Outpatients today without the luxury of having the notes available..." – I won't even go there.

Anyway, I ought to get back to the brief in hand. Please forgive me the odd literary meander. I remember reading *Dreams, Memories and Reflections* by Carl Jung as a teenager and loving the name of the book. The problem now is that I can't quite remember which is which, but you might get a touch of all three in the forthcoming pages!

Staring at screens, if allowed, can put a wall up when trying to communicate to the best of our ability. They have the same attraction as fruit machines – flashing screen messages, QOF and other reminders. The messages may well be 'urgent', such as "Mr X is in Reception and needs his prescription signing" (the joys of 'on-call', eh?) or reminders of blood pressure or bloods that need doing. Have I done the COPD review? They need their flu jab! Yes, all potentially important stuff, and can inject income into our struggling coffers, but surely the consultation process is paramount to our patient's wellbeing and future trust in us. We can address such issues if necessary at the end of the consultation, or even save them for another day.

I really don't think we should be caught screen watching when the patient is either coming in or leaving; they deserve better. It happens to all of us occasionally, especially as our internal focus and external interaction with our patient become divided, which is understandably often the case when we're trying to organise our minds into some sort of diagnosis, plan, etc. We have to be careful doing this as we can occasionally miss some golden nugget of information presented to us, or a non verbal cue offered our way. I may even apologise if I'm thinking too hard, and ask the patient to repeat what they just said.

When to enter the data is another matter. Usually I'd wait until the end of the consultation after our patient has left. This gives your mind time to bring all your thoughts together and make sure all bases are covered. I might also jot down anything that needs reviewing next time. Occasionally, rightly or wrongly, there may be so much information offered that I need to jot a few things down during the consultation. Often, if I do need to type during the consultation process, I'll let the patient know why. Something like: "It must seem really ignorant of me to do this, but I really need to remember everything you say, and I *am* listening"... Again, if you need to look at the screen, I'd suggest that you briefly share why you are looking at the screen with the patient. Something like: "Sorry for looking away; I'm just trying to get the exact details of what happened in the ENT department, and when they intend to contact you again."

Welcoming your patient in...

This is so important. It's worth remembering that the 'balance of power' will generally be perceived as leaning towards the clinician. They come into our room, on our terms. We appear to 'call the tune' and hold the information our patient is so desperate to gain. We literally hold the key to their future wellbeing. This can be really intimidating; they may also be somewhat nervous about discussing their most intimate problems, and even scared of what we might eventually diagnose. Doing whatever we can to alleviate these anxieties at the very start is paramount.

The first ten seconds sets the tone for the whole consultation. They need to know that you're interested, that you care, and that no other external issues are currently on your mind. This is one of the reasons the previously discussed 'head start' is so important. You already know to some degree about their situation, so there's no last-minute screen grabbing for information. Welcome them in, if possible with a smile! Look them in the eye, and make them realise that in the next few minutes you are there for them, and them alone. What to call patients can sometimes be awkward; I generally call them by their first names as I've known most of them for so long. If in doubt, I'll ask. I may have left a note in a previous consultation around how they like to be addressed. There seems to be quite a lot of folk who are actually known as their middle name. If you find out, note it down, and put it in the 'like to be known as' part of the registration screen. It can make such a difference. If they're officially known as Brian Eddie, but known as Eddie, then being called 'Brian' is already putting up some sort of barrier, and calling them 'Eddie' shows that you've taken note, and you care.

Caring…

If there's one thing to make obvious in the consultation, it's that you care, and that you'll do your very best for them. The rest generally falls into place thereafter. My hope is that most of you find my questioning how much you care vaguely insulting, but these levels can be variable at different times, on different days and situations. I think it's the caring and making a difference that makes our job so fulfilling, so it's a 'win win' situation. I'm sure most if not all of us went into this career for the purpose of helping people. Some of you may have fallen out of love with general practice for various reasons; external pressures, increased demands and constant change can sometimes make this role of ours a bit of a journey of survival. The role of GP partner is complex and multifaceted. Many GPs have taken on the roles of businessmen or women, managers, and so much more. I actually gave up my managerial role a few years ago. I soon realised that I was not really trained to be a GP partner in its entirety. There were serious issues with our practice manager at the time, the manager in whom I had put all my trust to make up for my own inadequacies in management, rather than take advantage of it. It was a lesson learnt, and I am far happier getting back to the job that I love: looking after and caring for the patients on my list. If there are those reading this who have 'lost that loving feeling', I strongly suggest taking stock of your working life and re-examining ways to get back to basics. Can non medical pressures be reduced? Having a top class manager to take pressures off you is a must. Just a tip from a wise head: find adequate ways of 'Managing your manager'. Trust is incredibly important, but don't take it for granted as an easy option…

'Mindfulness' is a bit of a buzz word which can be overused, but it may be a suggestion to clear your mind if possible for each of these fifteen-minute sessions, gaining an amazing level of job satisfaction by helping another human being. In fact, caring is the 'Pièce de résistance' of medical practice; the rest is merely garnish.

Allowing freedom to express

After making sure your patient feels as comfortable as possible in these odd-ish surroundings, it's time to let them tell their tale. I generally start with something like "So how can I help you?" although there is obviously a variety of options that you can develop to suit your style. An open ended invitation to express why they have come to see you will hopefully give the freedom needed to try and explain their issues in a non pressured environment. Responses to this tend to vary; on average I'd suggest around 2-3 minutes is reasonable. Some take considerably less time, and some potentially a lot more. Flexibility on our side of the table is a must, although the time may come where we may have to intervene and add a little 'control' into the proceedings. This 'free' time is so important, and deserves our total concentration. Eye contact is a must, and intermittent supportive gestures or words can be useful to help make them feel at ease. A simple nod may be enough, or even an "aha" to encourage them to continue. A quiet, unassuming "aha" rather than going full Alan Partridge, obviously!

At some stage we start to get a decent idea of where the consultation may be going. Towards the end of this free time, my mind starts to turn over. What am I thinking is going on? What might I want to do? Sometimes 'histories' can be complicated and certain parts unclear. Summing up your take on the story might be a good idea; hopefully this is when the patient's 'freedom of speech' is drawing to a natural conclusion, although there are times when you may need to intervene. This needs to be done subtly, apologising if necessary, but also making the point that you want to clarify their side of the story.

By now there may be definite questions that need answers in order for us to create a list of tentative diagnoses, as we mentally start putting some sort of plan together. Examination of some sort may be useful to further clarify the situation.

Examination

It may be a little challenging of me to suggest that examination to make our diagnoses is not quite as important as it once was. It is, however, still necessary, not only as part of our diagnostic armoury, but also to satisfy patient concerns. I can't remember how many times patients have said to me "I went to hospital and got a thorough examination"; the 'laying on of hands' goes back to the early days of medicine, and it does appear to be quite a reassuring process.

The COVID situation has got me thinking, however. As someone in the high risk category, I personally have examined far less than ever before, but with care – even more care than before – in the history taking, I feel I have treated my patients pretty well. Investigations are so easy to access these days. Whereas in the past abdominal examination, for example, was incredibly important, I know now that I can get an Ultrasound booked within a couple of days. I have spoken to three men with testicular swellings over the past couple of months. Previously, not examining would be totally unheard of. Even delaying a couple of days would worry me. So I'd examine, and even if they appeared to be something benign like epididymal cysts, I'd send for Ultrasound for total reassurance, both for me and my patient. During COVID I've gone directly to Ultrasound, and within a couple of days I've got my results to share. Bloods as well are easy to access – too easy, maybe.

Interestingly, the one examination that has been necessary has been chests. Discerning symptoms of chest infection versus heart failure, for example, is incredibly difficult without examination. If there's any suggestion, even 1 in 100, of cauda equina syndrome, you'd better get examining, and if not, send them to A&E! Legally speaking some examinations are paramount.

I'd also be wary of not properly assessing those at either end of our life spectrum, the very young and the elderly. Both groups are extremely vulnerable, making early diagnosis and treatment so important. I'm seeing less of those with simple self limiting conditions – fewer colds, earaches and the like – however, safely netting, as mentioned below, is so important in case the situation deteriorates.

I must admit there are times when I've felt uncertainty in consultations. Should I admit, or not? I think this child is absolutely fine, but... There are so many examples. Most decisions are fairly easy, and we're totally comfortable with them. Other examples might include whether to refer or not, or even whether a patient reaches the threshold for a 'two week wait' potential cancer referral or not.

Dealing with Uncertainty

In such cases of uncertainty we need to a) recognise the presence of said uncertainty and b) document both positives and negatives in history and examination fastidiously.

'Gut feeling' is something we talk about regularly. Something inside us tells us, despite what we see, that we're missing something, and things aren't quite what they appear. I'd suggest taking this seriously, and use this feeling to redefine your assumed scenario. Concentrate that little bit more. This 'gut feeling' is actually your bank of experience telling you that the normal patterns, the signs, symptoms and physical findings, do not quite conform exactly to what you are used to. Your initial thoughts may well be right, but listen to that internal voice – it's telling you something for a reason. Similarly, listen to patients' internal voices, particularly when their children are involved. Some parents can obviously overreact to their child being unwell, but they need to be listened to, and if you are a hundred percent sure, then offer reassurance with the proviso that there is an adequately large safety net if the situation changes, or if the parent fails to accept this reassurance you are offering.

Safety netting is massively important, but what does it mean? It means putting things in place in case things don't quite pan out how you hope. As GPs, we are the risk managers of the NHS. It's part of our DNA; we have to be good at it, otherwise every patient would end up with a barrage of investigations, and so many would be admitted to hospital. After all, every child with a cold could possibly have meningitis; every adult with diarrhoea could have bowel cancer, or those with coughs might have lung cancer. This is not an attempt to scare you; I'm just going on from the 'risk management' theme – there is a risk, no matter how small, and we need to be aware of it and prepare accordingly. This ought to be incorporated into the 'plan' we are, with the patient's permission, starting to build.

Building a plan

As I have discussed previously, at some stage in the consultation process we need to start putting a plan together. This obviously varies according to what the consultation is about. There are so many factors involved in this process, and I have included some of my thoughts about all sorts of things in this section as they would come under 'what can we do for our patient?'.

Once I've clarified what I perceive to be a reasonable way forward, I will start sharing with our patient. I've hopefully summed up the symptom presentations, giving them a chance to clarify any points still unclear. If it's a clear-cut diagnosis, I'll share my thoughts on what the treatment will be, and rough timescales over which improvement in symptomatology may be expected to occur. This is important; I don't want someone still coughing in four weeks, yet it might be 4-6 weeks before antidepressants start to work. If the diagnosis needs clarification, investigations or even referral may well be needed. It may be clear and obvious how to progress, such as blood tests or proceeding to X-ray. Often, however, it's not so obvious. There may be different potential pathways available. So how on earth do we choose? Ideally we'd like the pathway that is the easiest and fastest for our patient. What I often find is that the easiest can be the most cost effective, a factor in this day and age I feel we should all be aware of.

Health Economy

This is another of my stable of hobby horses. Having sat on numerous boards over my many years in health care, I realise we all have to play a role in looking after our amazing NHS's precious funding. There is a balance here, of course, between obsession around saving money which drove me away from certain political boards, and a personal responsibility to make every pound work its utmost to help our patient.

Maybe this doesn't sit too easily with you. I'll put some scenarios your way to form a basis of discussion.

I've held several political positions locally over the years; one I loved and learned so much from was sitting on our medicines management committee. At that time, the mainstay of the treatment of abnormal lipids was two-fold, Simvastatin and the new Atorvastatin. Forget that now Atorvastatin is the drug of choice, as those were different times. At that time, Simvastatin cost £1 monthly and Atorvastatin around £30 per month. The evidence at the time also leant towards Simvastatin with the massive Heart Protection Study. And yet some local GPs were using Atorvastatin as "each patient deserves the best I can offer". Of course pharmaceutical reps, who were prevalent 'advisers' at the time, were heavily promoting Atorvastatin. I visited some of these surgeries to try and discuss both the evidence and financial ramifications, but was largely dismissed. "It's not our job to discuss funding – we're just here for our patients."

There were no 'budgets' at the time for us to ponder over, and GPs' pens were running riot signing prescriptions (and referrals...) without any concept of the cost. We are now far better informed. The cost of medication is obvious to us within our IT systems; I'd also welcome more openness around the cost of other services. A few years ago as 'neighbourhood lead' I knew exactly what everything cost. Now I'm back working simply as a GP, it's sometimes difficult to find this information. What I'd really like to know is how much things cost, what the waiting times are, and even how easy it is for patients to get to the appointment.

I'd also like our hospital based consultant colleagues to have some sort of concept of what Health Economy means; after all, we're all in this together. As the 'commissioners' of care we in primary care have been handed the poisoned chalice of holding the purse strings, but I think all who key into services should be aware of their costs, and how precious to taxpayers NHS resources are.

Scenario – patient with back pain/sciatica

I've thrown this into the mix as it's common, and there are usually a large number of pathways available to go down. It can also show how things have changed for us over the years.

Let me take you back thirty years or so ago. Access to scans was limited to consultants only; even then it was rarely done as there were maybe only two or three scanners across a whole area. Typically, all patients with back pain were referred to an orthopaedic surgeon, and were seen maybe six months later. They were then referred on to Neurosurgery if there was a sciatic element (another six months) who arranged a scan, as they were the gatekeepers. The scan took another three months. If it showed a potentially operable lesion, it was booked in for surgery. If not, a referral to Physiotherapy was made, with a further wait of several months. This situation was hardly ideal for our poor patient, and awful for our health economy.

Now I have numerous options. Our PCN (Primary Care Network) has a musculoskeletal service, and the physiotherapists running the service will contact our patient within a week or so. I also have the choice of using a direct access MRI scan if there is possible nerve entrapment; if there is a potentially operable lesion, I can run it by a neurosurgeon. Our neurosurgical unit is quite a trek away, so I might ask them to look at the scan first. Why send my patient to Salford if I can get an answer while they are sitting at home? It's also worth discussing with the patient as part of the plan. Explain why you are involving a neurosurgeon. They may not want surgery. How many times have I seen letters from referral colleagues suggesting surgery is a possibility, but that the patient doesn't want it? If surgery was talked about as part of 'the plan', I probably wouldn't have wasted a) the patient's time or b) my precious resources sending them to visit a neurosurgeon, whose great skills are not actually wanted by our patient.

Other options include pain clinics. Some can be brilliant and holistic, some not. I have two options locally and I know which referral if necessary I'd prefer. It's also cheaper as it's a part of a community service...

Know what resources are available

If you're going to do the best you possibly can for a patient, you really do need to know what is available to use. You can be top class at consulting and have dream-like communication skills, but if your sole method of seeking advice is to do routine referral to the local hospital, your patient may be seriously missing out. I've no idea what may be available to you, my reader, unless you are working next door to me, but I'm sure you could find out.

I've even gone as far as asking my secretary to allow me to triage all locum referrals. It's not that I don't trust them, but more that I know what pathways may be available for me to key into for my patient. I've already used the back pain/sciatica scenario to discuss how different pathways can make a massive difference, often improving the patient 'journey' while also saving the health economy a small fortune.

Recently I triaged a cardiology referral. The patient had uncomplicated atrial fibrillation found on a routine ECG. If our locum's referral had been followed through, they would have waited for their cardiology referral then trouped up to the local hospital, struggling to park and then waiting a couple of hours, by which time the parking ticket would probably have run out... The cardiology consultant would probably have referred for hospital-based Echo, a hospital-based 24 hour tape, followed some months later by a further review. That's four trips to the hospital, with results and review in probably six months or so.

So what did I do? First of all I rang the patient. CHADS-VASC2/HASBLED suggested anticoagulation, so after discussion around stroke prevention and potential risks I started on Rivaroxaban 20mg daily straight away. That's six months' stroke prevention advantage for a start. I then referred for community-based Echo, and community-based 24 hour trace, both easily available to me. I then forwarded the results to our local cardiologist for 'advice and guidance' just to make sure that everything was in hand. The investigations took around four weeks altogether, and the advice and guidance came back the next day. I think you'll agree that this was so much better for the patient, and also vastly cheaper; advice and guidance I think is currently around £25 compared to £160 for an outpatient appointment.

It's worth investigating exactly which departments offer 'advice and guidance' locally; I think you may be surprised, especially now so many more hospital departments have realised post COVID how effective guidance, as well as telephone intervention, can be.

Other local interventions I love include our community 'extensivist' service, and recently added 'community matron' service. These are both amazing for those extraordinarily complex cases that you might need support with. I do find in the most complicated cases another set of eyes can help;

they also have far more time than me to get involved. Our 'community matrons' in particular are highly trained practitioners who can clarify the extent of physical issues as well as keying into social problems, and referring accordingly. These have been employed for our locality by our PCN – a great use of funding in my opinion. Since we've got these brilliant community services now, I rarely if at all refer to hospital based elderly medical or falls clinics.

Re falls, as well as the services above, we have a stunning community based 'urgent care team' that can respond within the hour if necessary. All it takes is a quick phone call for the linked social services, physiotherapist or occupational therapist to respond instantly if necessary. What a dreadful shame it would be to overlook using an option such as this locally.

If in doubt about any service, then picking up the phone and speaking to someone usually gets results. A recent example is with support for one of my patients with poorly controlled diabetes. He had been referred to our community based diabetes service by one of our practice nurses. A quick phone call and I had not only support and expert involvement almost immediately, but also our local diabetic specialist nurse's mobile number to hand for future reference! (I do love my extensive list of contacts in my phone! Cardiologists, gastroenterologists, rheumatologists to name but a few. I don't think they mind my annoying them too much... and if it gets a result for my patients I don't really care!)

There are so many more community based services I could talk about which offer support with the physical scenarios that are presented to us. Knowledge around local services offering holistic support is just as important. Being involved on Hattersley estate for all those years has helped my knowledge, but it takes effort. Last year I took a day's study leave to find as much as I could about what was going on in the community. I went to the local community hub and chatted to various community leaders. I spoke to the Citizens Advice Bureau adviser who visits Hattersley every Friday; I had a chat with a community development officer, and linked up with the local housing committee. I even visited a community gardening project, and learnt about walking clubs, 'casserole clubs' where folk chat while cooking, and 'Men in Sheds' for lonely men.

Luckily all such community services have been linked together for us, and it's incredibly easy to refer into our local 'social prescribing' hub via a single button in EMIS. Interestingly, in some circles 'social prescribing' seems to be frowned upon, and I'm not really sure why. Just recently I witnessed a Twitter (of which I am a massive fan) pile on, with so many medics complaining about the concept of social prescribing. I really can't see any problem with looking at other ways to advance a patient's holistic wellbeing. In our surgery we have engaged patients in a scheme to help other patients. They are termed 'patient champions,' and have done so much for the total care we as a surgery can provide. We have Tai Chi sessions in our waiting room (I took part in one session), a Parkinson's cafe, sessions where patients can chat while making sandwiches for the homeless. The list goes on.

'Integration'

'Integration' of services was being talked about a good few years ago. I think it came round as a result of financial need. There are obviously links. A couple of examples for your perusal: an elderly person is fit for discharge, but has deteriorated as a result of frailty or chronic illness, and sadly is unable to go back to their previous situation at home. The cost of a hospital bed which they occupy is around £550 per night. The cost of a suitable nursing home bed is around £200 per night, but social services have had their budgets slashed and are wary of picking up the bill, hence so often patients stay in hospital, which doesn't really help anyone. Making it a unified budget between health and social care would surely make sense for all concerned. Locally this has actually made a massive difference.

Another simple example: our elderly fall regularly on icy pavements. Sadly the council can't afford to grit the pavements properly, so they remain slippery. A fractured femur costs the health economy around £10,000. Putting a fraction of that money into preventing these falls surely makes sense.

Similar integration of primary care and hospital services are also moving rapidly, for everyone's benefit. There are too many examples of excellent integrative practice to list them all. Locally our diabetes services have moved into the community, and I was pleased to be clinical lead for diabetes during that process. We have teams giving intravenous therapy in the community, community physiotherapy services and a whole host of services being moved out of hospitals. Again, it's better for patients to stay at or near to home, and they tend to get a better quality of service for a more competitive price.

To be honest, I'd like to take this 'integration' a whole lot further. I still feel that communication is too often lacking between various clinicians looking after our mutual patients. I'm rarely called when my patients are in hospital. Tests are duplicated, medications are started that I've tried unsuccessfully in the past, and other meds stopped that were commenced for very good reasons. We need to talk more. This can also be the case when patients are seeing separate consultants for 'different' issues, and they rarely think of talking to each other. It's so important that we as GPs keep an eye on such patients. We are the central cog in their treatment wheel. It's not enough to relieve our responsibility totally as they are 'under the hospital'; we really need to keep our eye on the situation. I can think of three or four times over the years when I have sent emails or letters to consultants in different specialities asking them to 'join up' their thinking. I've even had patients under similar departments in different hospitals undergoing the same investigations in each. Why on earth in this day and age are our IT systems not integrated into one large, all-encompassing system? Surely this makes sense, and can't be too difficult to realise. I keep getting told this is 'on the horizon' but the horizon doesn't seem to be getting any nearer!

I would ideally like us to be somewhat more radical in bringing services into the community. It tends to be a given that consultants live in hospitals, and GPs in their surgeries. How useful would it be for me to be on a medical ward round discussing my patients with the consultant? With the history of trust coupled with access to our clinical records, surely it would be a winner? I'd love consultants to work with us more; we could learn so much of each other. Another bonus would be my knowledge of what services we have in the community, and also some background around what level of functioning we can hope to achieve, knowing as we do their recent history and home situation.

Mental health tips in our consultation- particularly depression

I always had an interest in mental health; it was my first 'SHO' job, and as I have already mentioned I worked as psychiatry registrar for a couple of stressful (I'm obviously lying...) years in Jersey. I really think our training in medical school was somewhat lacking. It was taught by hospital consultants in a hospital environment. I distinctly remember being given an hour to take a psychiatric history, and an hour to formulate a plan. I'm sure it was high quality teaching, but hardly set any of us up with the tools to treat mental health issues in primary care. I do have a weird memory of a hospital consultant ward round. There were about twenty of us, all sat in two lines with the consultant like the king at the end. The poor patients walked one by one through this line of assorted people. I did wonder whether it was the consultant's idea of flooding therapy... whatever it was, it hardly helped. (My mind drifts to another fleeting memory of medical student life in the early eighties, when all six medical students in a urology clinic were told to do rectal examinations on a single outpatient attendee – let's hope it has all improved!)

Getting back to my original train of thought about dealing with issues like depression in one of our fifteen minute slots, obviously we don't have the hours available so need to cut corners compared to hospital histories, but we can make a real effort to listen, empathise, formulate a diagnosis and move towards a plan, much like in previous paragraphs.

What I think is so important is to try and draw out what I believe to be a rather important diagnostic issue in such consultations, that being to define simplistically whether our patient has a depressive disorder or otherwise chronic unhappiness. Hopefully being empathetic will give our patient the confidence to tell their tale. Persistent lowering in mood may represent a depression, but I really need to know if this is a change from their normal personality. The concept of 'premorbid' personality, taught to us in medical school, is so important. If there has been a change, then a depressive disorder is more likely. It's often difficult to clarify if there were any causal factors, so trying to time this 'change' is really useful. Did the lowering in mood impact on the relationship, causing breakdown, or did the breakup impact on their mental state? After getting an idea of this, I'd tend to clarify whether there are any biological features of depression, such as loss of appetite, sleep disturbance and 'diurnal variation in mood', with mood typically being worse in the morning. Loss of concentration often also occurs. I used to ask if they can watch an episode of Coronation Street without losing focus, but nowadays I don't think even I could! I did once ask about Eastenders but soon thought better of it...

If I'm certain of the presence of a depressive illness, I may start to discuss depression and its management. The part around 'sharing the plan' here is so important. They may not have thought of it as a potential diagnosis, or even be aware of it as an illness as such. If anti-depressants need discussing at this stage, again it needs to be done carefully. There are often misconceptions around addictiveness, and these need to be addressed. It should be pointed out that their effect can take time, often an initial 4-6 weeks, but potentially even longer if the first dose used is ineffective. I'd probably also mention that treatment for at least six months is ideal, otherwise the beneficial effects of medication may be reversed. I have also written a leaflet for patients I diagnose with depression, as it is often helpful to share this with their nearest and dearest, and it is important to consolidate the main messages given. I tend to arrange follow-up appointments myself and actively contact them, as their short term memory and concentration may be affected by their illness.

This is very brief, I realise, but I seriously think we can be of massive help when it comes to depression. As I have said previously, caring and being perceived as being caring is paramount. Often these folk have spent an age worrying about themselves. Mental health issues are so difficult to live with. Sufferers show no obvious signs of illness to others around them, no plaster cast on their injured leg or shortness of breath to gain sympathy. Those close to them may even find it more difficult being around our patient; often irritability is a big part of depression, and they both may be struggling to get an insight into what is going on. We can help not only the person seeking help, making a potentially massive difference to them and their future, but also the relationships and lives of those affected by their friend's or relative's illness.

Medication reviews

We're often expected to do med reviews as part of a number of things in a consultation. The date for review has long gone, and here is our patient with his or her two or three issues they wish to discuss. The temptation is therefore to 'tick the box' at the end of the consultation, maybe with a cursory "Are you okay on your current meds?" We may get away with this if the number of medications is limited; Thyroxine for thyroid disease, and their recent bloods are fine; just inhalers, and they've had their thorough asthma review by one of our excellent practice nurses; diabetes with no complications. Our nurses have actually reviewed and are happy with their meds, but they don't do 'med reviews' as such. Anything more complicated and their medication does actually need properly reviewing. My suggestion is that anyone on more than six medications needs an appointment for the review alone. Often these days reviews are done by pharmacists who are a brilliant addition to our primary care team – personally I think every practice should have their own pharmacist.

Let's give a simple example of how detailed medication reviews can be useful, and how if they're not done properly things can go wrong. A patient with hypertension wasn't feeling too well. I noted they were on Ramipril, Amlodipine, Isosorbide mononitrate, Furosemide (I've finally stopped writing Frusemide..) Atorvastatin and aspirin.

Why Furosemide, I wondered for a start. Well, three years ago they had ankle swelling that didn't improve with simple measures, and the diuretic Furosemide was started at the suggestion of a doctor in A&E. Even my limited pharmacology knowledge had me staring at the Amlodipine, which I presume we all know can cause ankle swelling. So they were on a tablet for the side effects of another one. Blood tests showed their sodium was low (Hyponatraemic), which was probably why they felt unwell. The diuretic which they probably didn't need had caused this. Interestingly they apparently had two med reviews since it was started, and it wasn't picked up.

Let's look further into this patient's story. I noted IHD (Ischaemic Heart Disease) 2002, and 'Normal Angiography' in 2003. Going back through the hospital letters, they were started on Isosorbide Mononitrate, aspirin and Atorvastatin by the local chest pain clinic, but had a normal angiography after the diagnosis, and a letter from the consultant suggested 'no evidence ischaemic heart disease'. Really as well as putting the code for 'Normal angiogram' onto the system, the code for 'IHD' should have been removed.

So how should this be dealt with? Sometimes sorting out these problems can be challenging, taking time and probably a few follow-up appointments. I like to do things in a stepwise fashion. Ideally, we would like them off the Furosemide, Amlodipine, Isosorbide and aspirin, but we'd obviously have to go slowly, adding alternative medication for blood pressure as we go otherwise their blood pressure may go up. Re the Atorvastatin, I'd be tempted to take off also and treat for primary rather than secondary prevention in due course... Oh, and while we're at it, maybe sort the Problem Summary list and take off the IHD register...

I'm assuming those buying this book have an idea about the above medications and conditions. If not, and you're not actually in the health care trade, I'm really sorry. If you're a GP, however...

Before pointing fingers, this wasn't an actual case, but many such cases put together. But I hope you get the drift. Ideally look upon medication reviews as an opportunity rather than an irritation. You may think you are saving appointments by being a little too swift, but you're stacking up a whole lot of issues for the future.

This is even more important in the elderly, where the situation above could have all sorts of consequences: falls, head injuries and even fractured femurs. How often do we see elderly folk with so many meds, often all 'evidence based'? They may have had a cardiac event, and their blood pressures are low due to the ACE inhibitor or beta blocker. They may even be intermittently hypo as someone has been chasing QOF targets rather than treating the patient...

I love evidence-based medicine. My point, however, is that care should be given to when such evidence is applied. If the patient's holistic life situation is put at risk, then maybe evidence-based medicine should be put to one side. This is the art of general practice: treating each patient on their personal merits, and using 'science' and 'evidence' for their benefit, not simply as a knee jerk reaction to perceived medical need.

Pain

A lot of patients are on high doses of all sorts of medication for chronic pain. Again it's tempting to say in their review "Are you okay on the morphine?" and gloss over; however, addressing their chronic pain and over-medication is in everyone's interests. This can be challenging for so many reasons. "I need to reduce your morphine" will probably sound dictatorial, and will undoubtedly wind the patient up. As I've pointed out previously, caring, and, just as important, being perceived as being caring, is paramount if a situation like this is to be addressed.

We need to point out that while it seems comforting to have strong medication, the evidence shows overwhelmingly that it doesn't actually help symptoms. We also need to offer to treat the pain in better, more holistic ways, to make up for 'taking the pain relief away'.

Understanding the start of the pain and medication cycle is important. The patients aren't intrinsically 'addicts', but in a way addicts of our making. This is not a criticism; in years gone by we thought we were helping this group of patients function better by increasing their pain relief. It is more a plea to offer understanding and help, rather than a simple 'they're addicted to opiates'.

I generally start with this wonderful video by Live Active which is freely available on YouTube, called *Understanding Pain in less than 5 minutes*:

https://youtu.be/C_3phB93rvI

I'd strongly suggest having a look. I have it on my desktop and will often watch it with my patients. I also have the link to hand to send to our patient via AccuRX before I see them. (AccuRX is a brilliant recent innovation which I love. It enables health care professionals to communicate back and forth with texts, photos and files.) This video shows brilliantly how chronic pain is programmed into our brains, and that the initial process causing the pain is probably not now an issue. This is expressed in cartoon drawings, and is extremely powerful.

The forming of our plan, and sharing of it, is so important. Our agenda before the consultation may well include reducing the opiates, where the patient's was probably to increase. Here is obviously a massive source of conflict. The danger is therefore that we start building up protective battlements on either side of our 'agendas' before we've even started. The drawing of agendas together has to be the improvement of the patient's level of functioning, and the message that this is our aim as clinicians has to be made obvious. Maybe sharing the goal of improvement in functioning rather than cure might help. This was a massive message I took to heart when I chose to visit Salford pain clinic a few years back. Before my educational visit I saw my target as a GP as making folk better in all situations, and felt I was failing if I did not. Nowadays, I'm more: "If we can improve your pain by say 20% would that be helpful, and would it help you deal with life better?" Setting future goals in functioning may also help, such as "What would you like to be able to do that you cannot do now?"

Pain clinics can be useful, although I personally think they vary dramatically in quality. In my mind they need to be holistic, and if there is no psychological support my personal opinion is that they might not be worth using. It might be worth having a conversation with local mental health services – do they accept 'living with chronic pain' as a referral option? So often I seem sadly to find that referrals 'don't meet criteria'. Another hobby horse, but I won't go into that now!

Summing up presumed presenting issues

By this stage we've gathered information, and hopefully have an idea around what the main problems are and how they developed. Summing up symptoms as we perceive them can be very useful. This lets our patient know that we are listening; it also gives them time to reflect on what they have told us. Have they missed anything out? Is the story correct, or is there anything they need to clarify better? I would say there are no hard and fast rules as to where in the consultation process this goes. It can even be done more than once if the story is complicated. We can then be fairly sure we've gathered the relevant information, and move on.

Sharing the 'plan'

This is the time in the consultation where I become a bit of a salesman. I've got my ideas about where I want the patient's care to go, and I need to sell it convincingly. How you 'sell' depends on so many factors; if there is already a trust built up within the consultation (and hopefully before) it will be somewhat easier. It may be about what you think the differential diagnoses are, and how you are going to try and find out. If you think their symptoms are likely not to be serious, it's worth sharing, as this might be their main concern. Of course, never fully reassure if you're not totally convinced. You may be pushed into reassuring: "It's not serious, is it doc?" I'd simply be honest, with something like "I think it's unlikely, but there are some tests I'd like to do to rule serious stuff out".

After sharing this information, it's a must to give time for questions or even disagreement. After all, this is a shared plan of which both parties need to have a level of ownership. I'd tend to give some idea of time with the plan. If they need bloods, I'll book them myself so they leave with an appointment with our health care assistant, and also a time I'll be following up. It's so easy to do this, and again is a pointer that you're taking a personal interest in getting them sorted. Why bring in another layer of admin, increasing work for both the admin team and our patient? They can then leave with not only a proposed plan, but actual appointments to make sure it all falls into place. Sending patients out, or getting them to ring in for follow-up can be really irritating. How are they going to have faith in me when I tell them I need to talk to them in two weeks, if there are no appointments at the desk for yours truly for four weeks? I usually say when giving these appointments that I'm organising their follow-up personally as I don't want to lose them in the system which can, at times, be a little overly stretched...

Is that okay?

This is often my final gambit to dig out any issues they may be harbouring. The reply, or even the tone of the reply, can give so much away. "Yes, that's great" is obviously ideal, after which you can rest assured that you've hit the target to some degree. Hesitation in answering is a bit of a giveaway that things aren't quite 'okay'... If you do pick up that there are issues, it's worth spending a couple of minutes to find out why. Is it one final question they feel hasn't been asked or addressed? Is it that there is a hidden agenda that hasn't been 'outed' yet? You can always find out briefly, and offer to address in greater depth at follow-up.

So what can possibly go wrong?

Sorry to say, but quite a lot for numerous reasons. For a start, we're all human; some people's personalities we like, and some we don't. It's normal for us not to like everyone, and it's also okay that some patients might find you not to their liking. Don't take it too personally as it's totally normal for people to show a preference. We can find other people irritating for all sorts of reasons, and often it can be difficult to define what's actually behind this feeling. I think recognising when patients wind us up is potentially important in a positive way. A little reflection may find the reason why. Do you have difficulty controlling their consultations? Do you feel they seek advice then ignore it? Do you have difficulty defining their agenda? Is it that they always come in with the dreaded 'list' – or is it simply that you're used to solving problems, and their problems are particularly difficult to resolve? Understanding a little more about the relationship with this particular patient can only be helpful, and there are occasions when expressing the difficulties you are feeling can not only be useful, but also set the improved scene for future consultations.

I remember several years ago a particular young woman coming in; she was always challenging, and somewhat difficult to help. After a good few meetings I said: "I really want to help you as much as I can, but I do feel a certain amount of hostility towards me. Have I done or said anything to upset you?" She said nothing for a minute, and finally let on: "You're not the only person to have said that". We moved on to her response to stress and worry, and that she was often perceived as aggressive. She tended to be confrontational without intending to be. We agreed on a referral into our counselling services, and consulting with her was a lot easier from that day on.

Unfortunately not all challenging scenarios end this way – that would make life far too easy!

'Lists'

A brief word about the dreaded 'list' of problems. As GPs we tend to joke about it; dealing with situations like this does, however, offer a significant challenge. I've seen it so often over the many years I have been practising (one would have thought that after so many years practising I'd be quite good by now…)

The patient comes in. "I've got a few things for you, doctor, and I've written them all down so I don't forget." They then slowly take out and carefully unfold their sheet of A4. You can only see a lot of very small writing, and maybe the number '9' half way down the page. Where do you start? The whole process I've described throughout this book is just fine if there is one over-riding reason why our patient has come. I've heard doctors say that they'll only deal with one problem. I've heard others say they will go to two!

Rather than letting the patient go through every single line one by one, I generally first put it to them that dealing with so many issues at once will probably lead to no single problem being dealt with adequately, and that maybe they should be dealt with in order of perceived priority. If I can sort out one issue properly, what would it be? I then like to take a look at the list myself (trying not to grab it off them too quickly). I like to make sure none of the symptoms presented may be interlinked. What if number one is the abdominal pain, and number five is weight loss? Also, as ever, we may have different agendas with different priorities. Number nine might be chest pain...

One thing to remember is we can't please all the people all of the time; our goal as practitioners is generally to do what the patient needs rather than what the patient wants. Most times they are one and the same; other times we can convince them that a certain path is better for their long-term health. However there will undoubtedly be times when we cannot give them exactly what they are looking for. I found the most common issue can be around the requesting of sick notes when we feel it's probably not indicated. Often when patients have been on sick for a length of time, I will discuss the future and suggest that getting back to work would be to their benefit. Luckily, I have a 'working well' team who visit our surgery regularly; they help counsel patients with the goal of getting them back into the workplace.

Another problem can be when a patient wants a certain medication prescribing. For various reasons we don't think it's indicated. Pragmatism is sometimes called for, such as using short term anxiolytics in a crisis. Our job, however, is to do what we think is best for the patient's health, and we have to hold our ground. Despite doing our best to discuss why we can't go down a certain path, our patient may leave unhappy, and the doctor/patient or practitioner/patient relationship seems to suffer. Sometimes offering another appointment in a couple of weeks is a good idea, when hopefully the relationship can be rebuilt. Other times they will 'talk with their feet' and see someone else in the practice. I don't generally suggest this, as I feel I'm passing my issue to someone else, but there are times when second opinions can be useful. One thing I would suggest is taking extra care in documenting all things discussed and suggested. This may help another member of the team in future, and also make it totally clear what happened in the consultation if there were ever to be a complaint.

Complaints

Complaints can take various forms, from a slight unhappiness with some part of the care giving process, up to a fully blown formal complaint for 'malpractice'. I have a few pieces of advice here. I tend to contact the patient as soon as possible in order to defuse the situation. It may be uncomfortable, but I'd suggest it's a better way forward than letters going back and forth, often with building resentment on both sides. If a 'mistake' is obvious for all to see, I would tend to apologise, and mean it. Many years ago I gave an elderly patient penicillin, when the notes stated clearly that she was allergic. My problem was that I went on a visit armed with a brief summary, and the allergy was not on the said summary. She ended up in Intensive Care, but thankfully made it through. Her daughter was understandably extremely unhappy, and a letter of complaint duly arrived at our surgery. I rang her, apologised profusely, and arranged to meet up the next day. I was just honest – how could I not be? I changed the way summaries for visits were produced, and we worked closely together a couple of years later when sadly her mum died. She simply wanted to know what happened, and sought an apology which of course she got. "I'm sorry" can at times stop complaints in their tracks. Other times not so, but my advice is not to get angry, or take it to heart too much. It will almost certainly happen to every one of you reading this should you have long careers as I have. It doesn't mean you are any less of a clinician, and remember that. If you do seem to get a lot of complaints, it's well worth asking those around you why that may be – they may have an idea; and if they are really decent colleagues they will tell you, and you will accept their candour with thankfulness.

Remote consultations/COVID19

I've always thought telephone consultation is a useful tool to have. Knowing so many of the patients makes it that bit easier. However, pre COVID I still felt I would benefit from seeing up to 50% of the patients I called. I tend to get a lot of patients with mental health issues; I still think that seeing them face to face is far better if possible. It just seems that bit more personable, when building up a relationship really matters.

Given that, we have had to do our very best during this crisis we have at present to fulfil our patients' needs remotely. The current Secretary of State Matt Hancock has suggested that all appointments should be by video unless there is a compelling reason not to. I hope he has made some time to represent some of us in court if need be. He might have a point that we may continue to deal with more patients remotely, but I really don't think he should have an opinion on this; I think the decision should be ours and ours alone.

So, any tips to improve our remote consultations? I think accuRX is an excellent innovation that has come into its own during this crisis... Sometimes patients aren't able to take our calls; they may be working or busy. I often accurRX them, maybe ask how they are doing; maybe ask for pictures if there are skin issues.

Video consultations can be useful; however I have found that those most needing them are those at home, particularly the elderly. They may have issues using the technology; sometimes relatives can help with this, but that assumes they want their relative to be part of the conversation. I have found 'end of life' video consultations quite challenging, to be honest. During the COVID crisis the coroner is accepting video consultation as last time the patient was seen, making certification easier, and smoother for the bereaved families. I have done this on a couple of occasions over the last few months, and I'm pleased to say I think the patient's needs in both situations were met, and both families reassured by regular daily phone calls. As soon as things go 'back to normal', however, I shall certainly go back to visiting.

The bottom line is we have to make sure our patients are safe. Diagnoses of cancers have gone down during this crisis, for various reasons. Patients may not have presented as they are scared to seek help; clinicians may have cut some corners when consulting remotely. If you are telephoning or videoing, take your time, even more than face to face if necessary. Remember that you're not quite going to pick up on the non-verbal cues that you're used to. Also, the little nods, the 'ahas' I mentioned earlier that keep the patient reassured that you're listening and want them to continue, won't flow quite as well and may be perceived as a disturbance in their flow, as only one person can talk at once. I'm following up far more, to reassure both the patient and myself that they are improving and out of the woods.

I'm also erring on the side of safety. I've always prided myself on my antibiotic stewardship for example, and I think my standards have slipped a little. I'm probably more likely now to treat productive coughs, for example, compared to when I could reassure myself that their chest was clear.

My final thoughts on this is that yes, we will do more, and become more effective at, remote consultations. Patients are also becoming more used to this as a consultation medium. In the past, I've often heard at the desk: "I don't want Dr Hershon to ring me, I'd like to see him". Now so many are happy to be called, either on the phone or via video; they seem to realise that so much can be achieved, and it's not just a 'quick word'. In my mind, however, face to face consultations will always be our gold standard. After we're all vaccinated, and hopefully COVID is history, we will continue to consult remotely more than before, but the face to face scenarios will remain a massive part of the ideal consulting process.

Final thoughts

So that's about it from me. I hope you've gained a little from my thirty years at 'the coal face'. I've loved my job and never ever regretted what I do. I'm not saying there haven't been difficult moments. Our jobs can be stressful; any job with the demand we have to meet coupled with the massive importance of the decisions we make will always bring some anxieties. My personal advice would be to work hard, obviously, but look after yourself in your 'down time'. Keep a healthy work/home life balance, and try to leave any residual anxieties back at the surgery when you leave. Without that, longevity in our roles becomes a problem, and 'burnout' a real possibility. This is the path we have chosen, and surely no job could be as fulfilling. Done with the utmost care, each of these magical fifteen-minute slices of time can make untold improvement in those we have the privilege to serve. If I've given you one or two ideas you think might help the way you practise, or if I've even made you think a little about things you may otherwise not have done, then my time spent on this has been well worthwhile. Helping folk improve their health is surely the best job in the world. Enjoy your careers. Embrace the changes and challenges put your way, and simply do your best. No one could ask for more.

Dr Andy Hershon Mb ChB MRCGP

Follow me on Twitter @andyhersh

Printed in Great Britain
by Amazon